Relieve Pain Without Side Effects

You Can Be Pain Free, Naturally

Terry Lemerond
and
Jan McBarron, M.D., N.D.

The purpose of this book is to educate. It is not intended to serve as a replacement for professional medical advice. Any use of the information in this book is at the reader's discretion. This book is sold with the understanding that neither the publisher nor the author has any liability or responsibility for any injury caused or alleged to be caused directly or indirectly by the information contained in this book. While every effort has been made to ensure its accuracy, the book's contents should not be construed as medical advice. To obtain medical advice on your individual health needs, please consult a qualified healthcare practitioner.

Relieve Pain Without Side Effects

Copyright © 2021 by TTN Publishing, Green Bay, WI
www.TTNPublishing.com

All rights reserved. With the exception of Chapter 9 – Doc to Doc – and any excerpts as permitted under the United States Copyright Act of 1976, no part of this publication in any format, electronic or physical, wmay be reproduced or distributed in any form or by any means, or stored in a database or retrieval system without the prior written permission of the publisher.

Library of Congress Control Number:
Print ISBN: 978-1-952507-12-0
eBook ISBN: 978-1-952507-13-7

Editor: Michele Olson
Design: Jill Baker
Formatting: Alt 19 Creative

Printed in the United States of America

This book is dedicated to all the true health seekers in the world.

Contents

1. What Is Pain?...................................1
2. Natural Solutions to Extinguish the Fire of Joint and Nerve Pain 9
3. Back Pain..................................... 25
4. Perceptions of Pain 35
5. Cost of Pain.................................. 41
6. Conventional Medicine's Response to Pain 49
7. Natural Pain Relievers That Work............. 57
8. The Triple Superpower Botanical Combo for Natural Pain Relief............................ 65
9. Doc to Doc................................... 77

Key References 87

References 89

About the Authors................................. 97

More about TTN Publishing, LLC.................. 101

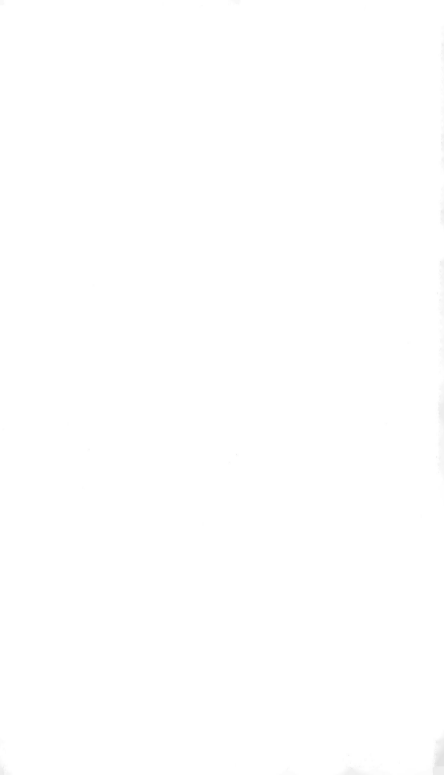

CHAPTER 1
What Is Pain?

If you are living and breathing, you have experienced pain. It's a part of life.

You put your hand on a hot stove and immediately, you pull it back. Your toddler does the same and that young body and brain already is wired to do whatever it takes to stop the pain.

We'll get to science in a moment, but it's important to understand from the beginning of this book that pain is a survival mechanism. Humans and animals (and perhaps plants) evolved to feel pain in order to be warned when something dangerous is happening so we can take action to stop whatever is causing the pain. If we didn't feel pain, we would probably walk into fires or off high cliffs. The memory of previous pain prevents us from putting a hand on the hot stove while the experiences learned from others prevents us from walking into the path of a speeding train.

Pain serves an important purpose: It alerts us when there is something wrong. With the hand on the hot stove, you know exactly what caused the pain. But what if you were feeling a sharp pain in your right side? That would probably prompt you to see a doctor or even go to the ER, uncovering the appendicitis that could turn deadly if not treated. Most of us know from experience that this kind of pain cannot be ignored.

The Science of Pain is Simple

With that hand on the hot stove, it is a pretty simple process:

1. There is a painful stimulus

2. Specialized nerve fibers in your skin called nociceptors send a message to the spinal cord and brain stem and then onto the brain

3. A sensation of pain is registered.

So, yes, indeed, pain is ALL in your head. Technically, the nociceptors, sometimes called "danger detectors," are the first line of defense in case of injury. It may sound strange, but these "danger detectors" are spread across all tissues of the body, acting as "eyes" of the brain that look out for threats. The nerves do not "feel" the pain, they just pass on the pain message so the brain can figure out its response. While the pain may be in your head, it is absolutely real. In a nanosecond, the brain sends back a message to pull back from the hot stove and your muscles respond.

Pain has many faces: sharp, stabbing, aching, dull, throbbing, stinging, pinching, burning or some combination of these. It can come and go, or it rears its ugly head only under some conditions, like when you sleep on your recently injured shoulder. You have probably experienced all of these in your lifetime, providing your brain with a library of possible responses when you encounter a painful experience.

We are certain you know someone with a high pain tolerance. Some people also have low pain tolerance. Think about a childhood friend who continued to play the softball game after a wrist-breaking slide into home plate. Then think about another friend who would cry over a skinned knee. Their perception of pain may have been the same even if the injuries were very different in severity. We do not know exactly why this is true, but we know for certain that pain is subjective and when someone complains of pain, take notice.

Acute vs chronic pain

There is acute pain, which is the brain's response to an assault: the hand on the stove, the stubbed toe or the thumb that you hit with a hammer. The injury happens, your body recognizes it, responds, and then initiates the healing process by triggering inflammation to increase blood flow, releasing healing molecules from nearby tissues and beginning the repair process. Usually there is some inflammation or swelling, a natural process to protect damaged tissue. Eventually, the injury heals, and life goes on.

Of course, we know that all pain is not caused by an injury. There are the moans and groans of aging joints, headache pain, nerve pain, and much more. Pain can be local—in one specific place or it can be general or even felt throughout the body.

Then there is chronic pain, pain that persists for three months or longer, possibly from an injury or some deterioration of the body's structure (most commonly joints), or it may have no known cause at all.

Any kind of pain is almost always accompanied by inflammation. Inflammation increases the sensitivity of the danger detectors, so over the long term, they may respond to situations that are not actually dangerous.

Think about the knee you injured as a young sports enthusiast. Over time, it healed. Sort of. But when you got into your 40s, you noticed how it ached on a rainy day. By your 50s, that dull ache was noticeable every day on your walk, and you'd occasionally ice it when it became truly painful. By your 60s, your doctor was recommending a knee replacement. That's chronic pain, caused by inflammation that, decades later, is still protecting that injured knee.

Chronic pain

Then there is what we'd like to call "chronic pain." You may or may not know the original cause, but the fallout over the years can become unbearable.

Translation

Decades of chronic pain can mess with your brain's response to pain, even if there is none there. Think about "phantom limb pain" that some people report after an amputation. They think they feel pain in the missing limb, even if that limb no longer exists.

This can happen when there is no missing limb. Your brain has become so accustomed to feeling pain that is sends pain signals for no apparent reason. It is a ghost of the original pain that your brain keeps repeating.

It is sometimes compared to the real engine trouble on your car as opposed to a check engine light that is on for no reason.

But that does not mean the problem, the pain, is any less real.

Referral

Long-term pain can also carry over to other parts of the body. If you injured your knee, you might be walking off-kilter eventually causing hip pain, back pain and even neck pain. Maybe it will even cause headaches. This is called referred pain.

Referral—pain in a part of the body that was not originally injured—can also be caused by nerve tissues firing like crazy, giving pain signals in places far distant from the actual problem spot.

Referral pain can be hard to diagnose for all these reasons.

Translation and referred pain are primary reasons for chronic pain and the disastrous pharmaceuticals that have led to the opioid addiction crisis. We will go into that in greater detail in Chapter 6.

Causes of Pain

There are numerous causes of pain. So far, we've mostly looked at pain caused by injuries and their long-term consequences.

But there are also other important causes of pain, including nerve pain, cancer pain, gut pain like you might experience from irritable bowel syndrome, and pain experienced after surgery. There are probably a nearly infinite number of other causes, including pain of unknown cause, the nemesis of health care professionals.

WHAT IS PAIN?

For the purposes of this book, we will be mostly focusing on musculoskeletal pain in joints, muscles, tendons and ligaments, and nerve pain caused by injury or disease.

By far the most common cause of musculoskeletal pain is the Law of Gravity. Just walking around our beautiful planet for a few decades puts a tremendous amount of strain on your joints and all the soft tissues that hold things together. In your lifetime, you have exerted enormous amounts of pressure on knees, hips, spine, and neck joints. Normal walking exerts three times your weight on your knees, so if you weigh 150 pounds, every step puts 450 pounds of pressure on your knees. Running is worse, exerting four times the stress on the joints or 600 pounds of pressure if you weigh 150. Gravity surely has consequences.

The support structure on our major joints does deteriorate over the years. The cartilage in knee and hip joints deteriorates and the pillow discs between spinal joints deflate. Not only do they deflate, but they can also press on nerves. Nerve pain is often caused by injury to the spine or brain, or diseases including diabetes, cancer, and shingles. All of these cause pain.

This book is meant for anyone who has ever had a minor or major joint injury, anyone who has had burning, numbing or tingling in fingers and toes, and anyone who wants to prevent these triggers for chronic pain. In this book, we will teach you to relieve chronic pain without side effects—how you can be pain free, naturally.

What You Need to Know:

- Pain is an evolutionary protection against damage from injury or a warning that something is wrong.
- Pain is transmitted to the brain by nerves. It is the brain that "decides" how to respond.
- Acute pain usually results from an injury or an illness that resolves itself in a short time.
- Chronic pain is longer term (three months or more) and is almost always accompanied by inflammation. It can last for decades.

CHAPTER 2
Natural Solutions to Extinguish the Fire of Joint and Nerve Pain

If you are of a "certain age," you have probably experienced joint pain. The echoes of injuries past or the grunts and groans that go along with changing position are signs of deteriorating joints, tendons, and ligaments. As we age, most of us are victims of the unrelenting lifelong pull of gravity.

Think of it this way: All the major joints, from neck to spine to hips, knees, ankles, elbows, wrists and hands, are cushioned by protective pillows called cartilage. Over a lifetime, injuries, exercise or lack thereof, occupational choices and gravitational forces break down those water and protein-filled cushions.

It is called "wear and tear" arthritis, scientifically known as osteoarthritis, and results in painful and swollen joints for 46% of all Americans. Those smooth cartilage cushions have broken down, torn or otherwise been damaged. Flattened spots create painful bone-on-bone contact and ragged edges can catch, causing more pain, swelling, and instability.

Nerve pain most commonly manifests as numbness, tingling, and burning sensations in the hands or feet. Affecting an estimated 20 million Americans, nerve pain, also called peripheral neuropathy, is most often a side effect of type 2 diabetes. About 70% of people with insulin-resistant diabetes have some form of nerve damage and pain. It can also be caused by autoimmune diseases like multiple sclerosis, irritable bowel syndrome (IBS), lupus, and others.

Compression of nerves like we often see in back pain, sciatica, and carpal tunnel syndrome is another major contributor to nerve pain.

Nerve pain is complex. It can also be caused by injuries, infections (shingles, for example), cancer, and chemotherapy. We will get back to that in a couple of pages.

Musculoskeletal pain

Let's look a little more at pain in joints, muscles, ligaments, and tendons, called musculoskeletal pain.

Trauma—in layman's terms, an injury—can be the beginning of an osteoarthritis cascade. That neck injury from a fender bender when you were 25 or the sports injury to your knee in high school or the sprained ankle in your 30s can eventually lead to cartilage deterioration that becomes osteoarthritis by the time you reach your 50s or 60s. More than half of all Americans over 65 have some form of diagnosed osteoarthritis. It is best to address pain completely at the outset if you can.

The deterioration triggered by an injury or by overuse does not usually cause immediate osteoarthritis, although it can. Serious joint damage is not unknown in younger people, especially in athletes who have repeated sports and overuse injuries. About 7% of people with osteoarthritis are between the ages of 18 and 44.

Conversely, couch potatoes beware: Not using your joints can also cause dramatic joint deterioration as can poor posture and repetitive movements like keyboarding or gaming, which is also a cause of compression nerve pain like carpal tunnel syndrome or sciatica. Obesity is a major factor in osteoarthritis because of the extra impact on joints, especially knees.

As we age, the incidence of osteoarthritis increases every decade. By the time we reach 70, most of us have some degree of osteoarthritis. Knee pain is the most common type of osteoarthritis in older people.

How does osteoarthritis feel? It has been described in numerous ways:

- Radiating pain
- Stiffness
- Loss of flexibility
- Tenderness
- Grating
- Locking
- Burning
- Swelling
- Instability

Treatment

Arthritis is often treated with exercise (this may seem counterintuitive, but movement seems to help lubricate stiff joints) and physical therapy. Joint replacement surgery, a painful major surgery, is often the best solution modern medicine can offer for relief in the face of severe osteoarthritis.

NSAIDs (nonsteroidal anti-inflammatory drugs like ibuprofen, naproxen, and prescription drugs like Celebrex, Voltaren and others) can offer relief in mild to moderate cases, but they have serious side effects like gastrointestinal pain, increased bleeding, allergic reactions, and high blood pressure.

NSAIDs (nonsteroidal anti-inflammatory drugs) can cause serious toxicity problems that require hospitalization for as many as 200,000 Americans each year and kill as many as 20,000. Yet 60 million of us use them regularly and doctors still happily prescribe them.

Sadly, highly addictive opioids have been commonly prescribed to treat osteoarthritis pain in an unknown number of patients with severe osteoarthritis, contributing to the national epidemic of addiction, overdose, and death from these terrible drugs.

Nerve pain

There are two types of nerve pain:

Remember in Chapter 1 how we talked about the nerves transmit pain messages to the brain? Sometimes, due to injury or disease, the nerves send pain messages to the brain nonstop. This is called nociceptive pain, pain in some part of your body that is transmitted by the nerves. For example, if you stub your toe or have an inflamed appendix, the nerves start sending excited messages to the brain that there is something wrong. This alerts the brain to send a normal pain signal that requires your attention.

Nociceptive pain can be somatic in response to an injury or visceral in response to nerve signals from the body's internal organs. It produces pain related to the cause of the stubbed toe or the abdominal pain from that inflamed appendix.

Neuropathic pain is long-term pain signaling there is damage due to a direct injury to the nerves like a pinched nerve or a disease that creates nerve damage like diabetic neuropathy or shingles. Neuropathy produces pain usually described as shooting, burning, tingling or numbing.

Treatment

The first line of treatment for nerve pain is much like that for osteoarthritis. Of course, if the nerve pain is caused by something like an inflamed appendix, immediate surgery will resolve the issue. Longer term nerve pain is usually treated like arthritis with NSAIDS and over-the-counter and prescription anti-inflammatory medications. Mild to moderate nerve pain may come and go, so these drugs can be effective.

Physical therapy, electric nerve stimulation or surgery may also offer relief.

Some sufferers of chronic nerve pain are given antiseizure drugs, like gabapentin (Neurontin) or pregabalin (Lyrica). Antidepressants like Cymbalta or Effexor may also address the pain itself. All of these can have serious side effects including liver failure, hallucinations, and low sodium that can appear like the symptoms of a stroke, seizures, labored breathing, aggressive behavior, and memory loss.

Opioids, including oxycodone, have become all too common drugs of choice to address the severe pain of neuropathy. We'll go into this more in future chapters, but it's important now for us to recognize the terrible toll these highly addictive drugs have taken, even when used for legitimate medical reasons.

There is Hope

It all sounds pretty grim. But there is good news: It's not a downhill spiral! There is a well-researched, natural and safe approach that offers widespread relief for people with all levels of joint and nerve pain.

Highly absorbable formulations of curcumin (*Curcuma longa*), *Boswellia serrata* (also known as frankincense) and black sesame seed oil (*Sesamum indicum*), botanicals widely used in the Indian Ayurvedic medicine tradition, display strong and immediate pain relief through their anti-inflammatory and antioxidant powers. Each of these three unique and synergistic botanicals individually treats and reverses the underlying causes of joint and nerve pain— deteriorating cartilage and nerve inflammation, unlike conventional treatments that merely address pain. Together, they have the synergistic power to relieve pain like no other combination.

Let's look at them individually.

Curcumin

If you love curry, you are familiar with curcumin, the active ingredient of the large-leafed turmeric rhizome (stem of the plant found underground) that gives curry powder its golden color. While curcumin is an ingredient of turmeric, it is tremendously concentrated and, therefore, vastly more powerful medicinally than plain turmeric. Here is an easy way to remember: Turmeric is a spice and curcumin is a medicine.

The Research is Impressive:

Reduce Inflammation: Biological indicators of inflammation were reduced by as much as 99% with curcumin, offering almost complete relief for chronic pain sufferers and providing powerful promise for prevention and treatment of other diseases caused by inflammation.

Cartilage Regeneration: Not only does curcumin help reduce the inflammation, but it also actually helps prevent the breakdown of cartilage. It prevents arthritis from developing or worsening, as shown by Canadian researchers. At least one study shows that curcumin can help build new cartilage cells, reversing what was once thought to be an incurable, degenerative disease.

Pain Relief: An Italian study showed that people diagnosed with knee osteoarthritis were able to reduce their need for NSAIDs by 63% when they took curcumin. As a welcome side effect in this study, it was discovered that curcumin produced a 16-fold reduction in participants' blood levels of CRP, the protein that indicates high levels of inflammation, which also predicts a high risk for a heart attack.

Rheumatoid Arthritis: A landmark 2006 study from the University of Arizona takes the idea of inflammation a step further with the finding that curcumin might prevent rheumatoid arthritis, an autoimmune disease that causes severe joint pain. Another study showed that curcumin was at least as effective as two commonly prescribed prescription pain relievers for rheumatoid arthritis.

Boswellia

Boswellia serrata, also known as Indian frankincense, extracted from the boswellia tree, has been used for centuries in Asian and African traditional medicines to treat inflammation.

Not only has boswellia been used to treat pain effectively without side effects, research confirms that this powerful anti-inflammatory can also prevent cartilage from degenerating. There are four acids in boswellia's resin that have been scientifically confirmed as anti-inflammatories, but Acetyl-11-keto-boswellic acid (AKBA) is thought to be the most powerful.

Here is the Research:

Reduce Pain and Swelling: A study published in the journal *Phytotherapy Research* in 2019 confirmed that boswellia safely reduced pain and stiffness in people with knee osteoarthritis. This confirms the pivotal 2003 Indian study that showed boswellia reduced inflammation and increased flexibility and walking time in people with knee osteoarthritis. What's more, boswellia reduced knee pain by more than 70% in subjects in a 2011 Indian human trial. A few of them with shoulder osteoarthritis got complete relief, plus another Indian study confirmed that boswellia "significantly reduced" the degeneration of knee cartilage, something scientists once believed was impossible.

Rheumatoid Arthritis: Several studies show that boswellia reduced joint swelling in patients with rheumatoid arthritis, an autoimmune disease. Probably the most exciting research from Germany in 2019 confirms that boswellia actually slows or even stops the autoimmune process by calming down the overblown immune response and reducing the numbers of inflammation-causing leukotrienes.

Nerve Pain: Remember those nociceptors, the nerves that carry pain signals to the brain? What if there was a safe botanical that blocked those pain signals? Well, there is, boswellia! Animal research published in 2017 in the journal *Evidence Based Complementary and Alternative Medicine* shows that boswellia blocked neurological pain receptors, binding to the opioid receptors in the brain safely and without addiction. We all know about the terrible opioid epidemic that has resulted in countless deaths and suffering, much of which began as legitimate treatment for pain. What if a safe and effective herbal could produce pain relief without addiction? Boswellia can.

Black Sesame (*Sesamum indicum*) Seed Oil

This Ayurvedic mainstay has unique properties that make it a powerhouse addition to our anti-pain cocktail.

Most of the research on black sesame seed oil's pain-relieving benefits confirms its powers to stop osteoarthritis and rheumatoid arthritis before they even begin, making it a wonderful ally in treating acute pain and preventing chronic pain.

It is a strong antioxidant that helps reduce cell damage caused by free radical oxygen molecules. An accumulation of free radicals in your cells act almost like rust on a metal surface, leading to inflammation and disease. Not only that, but black sesame seed oil can even reverse the cell damage caused by those free radicals.

Another unique and exciting property of black sesame seed oil is that it has been scientifically proven to help regenerate deteriorating tissue, including the cartilage cushions in joints. Even just one of the compounds in sesame seed, sesamin, can help increase type II collagen and prostaglandins and prevent the breakdown of beneficial fatty acids that keep joints healthy and stop painful damage before it can deteriorate.

Sesame seed oil contains healthy fatty acids that have been shown to stop joint inflammation, reducing the activity of TNF-a, inflammatory proteins called cytokines that are responsible for much of the damage caused by the inflammation that triggers various types of arthritis.

In clinical research, supplementation with sesame seed has been shown to reduce inflammatory markers, pain scores, and symptoms in patients with knee osteoarthritis.

In another unique function of sesame seed oil, a Taiwanese animal study confirmed that it is equally effective against nerve pain like sciatica.

Additionally, sesame seed oil appears to help other nutrients absorb more effectively, having a synergistic effect on, and helping concentrate levels of vitamin E tocopherols, vitamin C, and vitamin K—all of which have their own antioxidant and anti-inflammatory powers.

Other general research with sesame seed has found that it helps control the ratio of omega-3 and omega-6 fatty acids, helps balance cholesterol levels and has overall immune, cardiovascular, and DNA-protective actions.

Double Superpower

Researchers wanted to know what would happen if they combined curcumin and boswellia. They were pleasantly surprised to learn that the two had a powerful pain-relieving effect.

The study published in *BioMed Central Complementary and Alternative Medicine* yielded impressive results. The synergistic effects of the two botanicals meant much more pain relief for people between the ages of 40 and 70 with osteoarthritis. Study subjects were able to perform much better on physical performance and pain level tests when they took 500 mg of curcumin BCM-95, a highly absorbable formulation, and 150 mg of Boswellia three times a day for 12 weeks.

Even more impressive, the safe and side-effect free combination therapy was just as effective as the prescription NSAID Celebrex, which carries increased risk of heart attacks and strokes and increased risk of death from both.

Triple Synergy!

So then, imagine what would happen if you combine curcumin, boswellia, and black sesame seed oil? That is exactly what researchers wondered in a groundbreaking 2020 Indian study that concluded that the botanical trio worked just as well as acetaminophen, just as fast, eased the emotional trauma of pain (more on that in coming chapters), all without the potentially life-threatening side effects that come with the use of acetaminophen. In fact, the three ingredients combined worked much better than each individual ingredient taken separately.

Researchers found that pain had almost disappeared within six hours, approximately the same time frame as with acetaminophen, again without side effects that range from gastrointestinal distress and ulcers to heart attacks, strokes, or death from liver failure.

If you had that sprained ankle or burned hand, wouldn't you prefer the safer and equally effective alternative?

Wow! In our minds, there is no question that a safe and effective triple combo is an obvious choice!

WHAT YOU NEED TO KNOW:

- Osteoarthritis, chronic inflammation of the joints, affects millions of Americans, most of them over 60 and is a significant cause of disability in the United States
- Nerve pain is a common side effects of diabetes, but also caused by injuries and a few other diseases that affects 20 million Americans
- These types of pain are often treated with powerful prescription drugs, including opioids, which can cause addiction, heart attacks, strokes, and death.
- Curcumin, boswellia, and black sesame seed oil individually have been scientifically demonstrated as safe and effective ways to treat musculoskeletal and nerve pain and to help regenerate deteriorating cartilage.
- In combination, absorbable curcumin, boswellia, and black sesame seed oil are powerful synergistic weapons against acute joint and nerve pain as well as the longer-term pain of osteoarthritis.

CHAPTER 3
Back Pain

Back pain is a part of life in Western society. Most of us sit in chairs in front of screens all day long. We spend evenings on the couch in front of the television.

Our exercise habits are pathetic! Fewer than 5% of American adults exercise 30 minutes or more a day, says the U.S. Department of Health and Human Services. Our kids are not doing much better with only one-third engaging in some kind of exercise on a daily basis, according to the President's Council on Sports, Fitness and Nutrition. In the last 100 years, since the invention of the automobile and mass transit, we have spent an unprecedented amount of time sitting. We're suffering for it.

What does this have to do with back pain? Everything!

Our ancestors were on their feet most of the time. Cave people hunted and gathered. Agrarian societies worked the fields. Even during the Industrial Revolution, most people performed physical labor for most of the day. Yes, life was hard, and, yes, lifespans were shorter, and our ancestors suffered and died from many diseases that thankfully do not exist today. But chronic back pain was rare largely because we were an active society.

Today, the World Health Organization estimates that 70% of residents of industrialized nations suffer from some kind of back pain. Other experts say that virtually all of us in the world will have back pain at some point in our lives.

There is acute pain—caused by an injury that heals in time and chronic pain that goes on and on, for months, years, even decades. Sadly, most acute back pain eventually morphs into the chronic category. This is true not only because of inactivity, but also because of the continuous pull of gravity on joints and soft tissues and the wear and tear type of arthritis caused by tiny injuries that may heal in the short term but take their cumulative toll over time.

Back pain is two-fold: musculoskeletal pain and nerve pain. Take a look at Chapter 2 again for a refresher on the differences between the two major types of pain.

Anatomy of Back Pain

Here is a brief anatomy of back pain:

The spine is a series of joints. It is literally the support structure of the human body. The s-shaped spine protects the spinal cord that runs through the 24 (depending on how they are counted) bony vertebrae in adults, almost like an electrical cord. That spinal cord has a network of 31 nerve pairs that branch out from the vertebrae These nerves, that control sensation and movement and a variety of involuntary nerve functions, act like telephone lines to the brain, which emit a response to the messages carried by nerves. The brain might simply tell the body to move, the head to bend forward or the legs to walk, all thorough signals sent back through spinal nerves. The brain might also tell the spine to respond with pain through those nociceptor nerves.

The vertebrae are the infrastructure of the spine. These bony structures protect the spinal cord. Each of the 24 vertebrae is cushioned by a donut-shaped, fluid-filled structure called a disc. Think of it as a jelly donut. These discs are the suspension system of the spine, tough as radial tires on the outside with a spongy interior that acts like a shock absorber to keep the vertebrae from banging together or the nerves from becoming entrapped. Sometimes discs rupture, deflating the "tire." Sometimes the weakened disc structure bulges.

It is relatively easy to visualize the damage that happens when those discs deteriorate because they dry out from age or because of old injuries. Vertebrae grind against each other, causing pain. Without their cushioning discs, vertebrae press on those branching nerves, transmitting pain messages broadly to the brain, most often resulting in pain in the legs and buttocks, a condition known as sciatica. Misaligned vertebrae and deteriorating discs can also expose the spinal cord itself to damage.

Osteoarthritis can also cause bone spurs to form on the vertebrae, destabilizing the spinal infrastructure or adding to misalignments and nerve entrapments caused by deteriorating discs.

Low back pain has huge costs. We will go into this more in Chapter 5, but let it suffice for now to say that back pain is the leading cause of disability throughout the world with enormous costs in human suffering as well as in lost wages and productivity.

Conventional Medicine

Conventional medicine has exceptionally poor results in treating pain. Diagnosis is difficult for a variety of reasons, primarily because chronic pain creeps up on the sufferer and the shifting infrastructure of the spine can make imaging difficult.

Similar to other types of joint pain, initial treatment usually involves NSAIDS and all of the attendant terrible side effects they can cause. As the patient's condition deteriorates, as it almost inevitably does, there are options for surgery, injectable steroidal pain killers, and more and more serious and addictive pain-relieving pharmaceuticals.

Here's why all of these fail, generally leaving the person in even deeper pain:

Surgery: There are several types of back surgery, all of which have at times been called "placebo" or even "sham" surgery to relieve pressure on nerves, remove damaged disc tissue or even to attempt to "re-inflate" the disc.

Even Harvard doctors warn against fusion, the ultimate back surgery in which two or more vertebrae are fused together, ostensibly stopping the pain.

> "It's a major operation that often fails to offer a lasting solution," says the June 2014 Harvard Medical School newsletter. "As a result, fusion has become the poster child for expensive, risky and unnecessary back surgery. Despite that, the number of fusions has risen sharply over the years."

> "...men with aging spines should be wary of fusion and its false promises," says Dr. Steven Atlas, an associate professor of medicine at Harvard Medical School. "Based on the evidence, the indications for fusion are few and far between, but that doesn't stop surgeons from doing them or patients from getting them."

Epidural Steroidal Injections: Doctors will often recommend epidural steroidal injections in the joint spaces to relieve inflammation and hopefully to relieve nerve pain. Generally, the relief can last three months if the drug is injected in precisely the right place. At best, these injections last about three months on the notion that relieving the inflammation may allow healing to take place and longer-term pain relief.

These can be dangerous for a variety of reasons, says a Mayo Clinic newsletter, including that the drug itself (usually cortisone), can weaken the vertebrae and nearby muscles, worsening the condition. They do not address the underlying causes of the back pain. The more injections a patient receives, the greater the possibility of side effects, including high blood pressure, diabetes, and obesity.

Pharmaceuticals: When NSAIDS fail, physicians increasingly turn to pain relief from drugs, most often opioids. We are now becoming painfully aware of the health-destroying nature of these drugs, including their high rate of addiction, overdoses, and death.

All of these are focused on stopping or managing the pain rather than addressing the underlying causes of the pain.

It all sounds pretty grim, right? It is. But, as you might imagine, this book provides a safe, natural and effective answer.

Curcumin, Boswellia, and Black Sesame Seed Oil to Relieve Pain Without Side Effects

What if there were natural ways to stop back pain *and* address the underlying causes?

All three of our superpower ingredients are well-researched anti-inflammatories, so it goes without saying that they can all relieve the inflammation caused by the structural damage to the spine and its nerves. They also stop the further damage that inflammation can cause. Simply reducing inflammation may sometimes provide permanent pain relief, but most often it does not. The bulging or herniated discs, bone spurs, and nerve compressions cause new inflammation.

Here's some tremendously exciting news: Curcumin and black sesame seed oil not only reduce the inflammation that causes pain, but it can also help rebuild disc tissues and strengthen the lower back. Wow!

In a 2017 animal study, researchers at the University of Virginia showed that curcumin can help the body generate new disc tissues, repairing ruptured discs.

Chinese research published in 2018 confirmed the pain-relieving properties of curcumin of the severe pain caused by nerve injuries, even though they didn't determine how it works, and earlier Chinese research confirmed that curcumin blocks the pain signals transmitted by the nerves and stimulates the brain's opioid (pain relieving) receptors without the use of dangerous drugs.

Boswellia has primarily been used as a pain management tool for back pain, largely because of its powerful anti-inflammatory effects.

Black sesame seed oil has the additional benefit of helping rebuild damaged tissue and soothing nerve pain like you'd have with sciatica, a painful condition when "flat tire" spinal discs press on nerves.

We know that the combination of curcumin, boswellia, and black sesame seed oil exponentially increases relief from osteoarthritis pain. The same is true of the combo for back pain. What's more, in addition to relieving existing inflammation, boswellia is believed to protect damaged tissues and stop the formation of leukotrienes, fatty molecules that start the inflammatory process.

A study comparing a combination of the curcumin and boswellia to the generic celecoxib (one brand name is Celebrex®) found that they relieved osteoarthritis pain for 64% of participants versus only 29% in the drug group.

Additionally, more people in the botanical group could walk without pain compared to the drug group! The message here is that the triple combo enhances each other's capabilities to reduce pain and the tissue-damaging inflammation that causes pain. When you use them, you are not just "covering up" the pain signals your body sends out, but rather helping your body to heal.

What You Need to Know:

- Almost everyone will experience back pain at some time, and it becomes chronic for millions of Americans.
- Conventional medicine treats back pain with drugs that have serious side effects, steroid injections that can be extremely dangerous and surgeries that are usually ineffective.
- Curcumin, boswellia, and black sesame seed oil have individually been scientifically validated to relieve back pain naturally, without side effects.
- Combined, the three have been shown to work synergistically to stop the tissue-damaging inflammatory process and even to help rebuild damaged disc tissue.

CHAPTER 4
Perceptions of Pain

Pain is subjective. One person might report "great" pain from a bee sting while another might barely notice it. Another might find a burn "nearly intolerable," while another dismisses it as "nothing."

The perception of pain depends on the complex pain stimulus-nerve perception of pain-brain response to pain axis we talked about in Chapter 1.

Remember the nociceptors, those nerve endings that are the first warning that something painful is happening?

Those nociceptors are everywhere in your body—skin, muscles, joints, and organs. When those nerves send signals to the brain at lightning speed, there is a response. Your brain receives the messages and tells the muscles to remove your hand from the hot stove or warns you that something is wrong with your appendix. These messages are complex and tell the brain where the pain is and how strong it is. Nociceptors are also specialized and can transmit several different types of signals to the brain:

- **Thermal**: Sense extreme hot or cold
- **Mechanical**: Transmits stress or strain as on a muscle or other soft tissue, like a tendon or ligament. Think about the time you accidentally did the splits or that dull headache that is plaguing you and you'll get the idea. It is also the way joint pain is transmitted, not necessarily as a sharp pain indicating an injury, but a dull ache and stiffness that confirm the injury has been around for some time.
- **Chemical:** Response to chemical stimuli, similar to what happens when you eat a habanero pepper.
- **Silent:** Response to something happening in an organ, possibly the first indication your appendix is flaring up or your heart has a problem if you are having abdominal or chest pain. Silent pain may manifest as a dull ache or a simple feeling that "something isn't right."

These four main types of pain signals can also occur in combination.

Pain Threshold and Pain Tolerance

You have probably heard the term "pain threshold." This means the minimum stimulation that causes you to register a sensation as painful. It is a very subjective measurement since all of us are individuals and all of us have differing concepts of and responses to pain. The most common test of pain threshold is to immerse your hand in a pan of ice water and measure the amount of time it takes for your brain to register the cold sensation as pain. Pain tolerance is measured when the pain of the ice water becomes unbearable.

Other tests measure response to pressure (a pin stick) or even an electrical shock. These are actually more easily measurable than the ice water because it's really hard to scientifically standardize the exact temperature of the ice water.

An interesting online experiment was conducted by the DNA testing company, 23andMe. Participants shot their own YouTube videos of their home trials with the ice water experiment. Most people began perceiving pain in less than 30 seconds. The hardiest of the bunch were able to stick with the pain for three minutes—a measurement of their pain tolerance. Instructions directed participants to have someone with them to time their endurance, perhaps adding a little element of bravado that might not have existed if they were alone.

Gender, hair color, and even dominant hand all play a role in determining pain threshold. This sounds a little wacky, doesn't it? Studies have shown that, in general, men are more pain tolerant than women. Natural redheads are less pain tolerant than people with other hair colors. You will tolerate pain better in your dominant hand (right hand if you are right-handed).

We also know that genetics play a role in how we respond to pain meds.

Why? There are some theories, but no one knows for sure.

Age is also a factor in pain perception as is social isolation in the opposite direction. Elderly people generally have a higher pain threshold, maybe because they have experienced pain over a decades-long lifetime. Socially isolated people tend to have lower pain tolerance, suggesting that our friend and family relationships help us to endure pain we might not be able to endure alone. Redheads may have a genetic cue called the melanocortin 1 receptor that makes them more sensitive to thermal pain and resistant to numbing agents like lidocaine.

Stress, past experience, and expectation are all major factors in perception of pain. Anticipating that something painful is about to happen can be stressful, especially if you have experienced it in the past. If you have had a painful dental procedure, for example, you would naturally be squeamish about undergoing another one.

Coping Mechanisms

So, you had that bee sting or broken leg or burned hand and it hurt. A lot. It's unclear whether there is a physical or psychological coping mechanism that eventually kicks in when pain becomes chronic. The pain of that sore knee may have seemed excruciating when you first injured it, but, as the cartilage deteriorates and the bone-on-bone pain becomes chronic, many of us find ways to live with it.

Does that mean the pain disappears? No. Not at all.

Researchers are not sure, but it is possible that those nociceptic nerves become a little jaded or weary of sending the same signals over and over. It is also possible that the brain stops recognizing the nociceptic signals as pain. That's where our understanding becomes a little foggy. Maybe people with chronic pain "retrain" their minds to neutralize the perception of pain. This may be conscious or unconscious.

Some people can successfully control or minimize pain consciously with "mind over matter" techniques like biofeedback, relaxation, breathing exercises, and cognitive behavioral therapy to distract them from the pain or to "compartmentalize" pain, meaning they mentally block it.

In conclusion, it is fair to say that we all experience pain in one way or another, that pain is individual and that we have some ideas, but we really don't know why some people experience pain in dramatically different ways than others.

What You Need to Know:

- Individuals respond differently to pain.
- Pain threshold is the level at which an individual's brain interprets a stimulation as painful.
- Pain tolerance is the point at which the pain perception become intolerable.
- Gender, dominant hand, living situation, and even hair color are factors in pain tolerance.
- Some techniques can help physically or psychologically to neutralize pain.

CHAPTER 5
Cost of Pain

Pain immobilizes us, not only physically, but emotionally. Just think about the last time you were in pain: a debilitating migraine, a burned finger, a sprained ankle. It is nearly impossible to think about anything else.

The mental stress and psychological effects of pain can be just as severe as the pain itself.

It can cause you to be cranky and irritable, that's for sure. As the pain continues, you may feel anxious, depressed, angry, misunderstood, and demoralized.

It is interesting that the experience of short-term and long-term pain is, of course, variable and individual, but it is also dependent on a variety of factors you might not have considered:

- Age
- Gender
- Culture
- Ethnicity
- Spiritual beliefs
- Socio-economic status

- Emotional response
- Support systems

The cycle of pain and emotions is interrelated, eventually creating a vicious circle. For example, if you are anxious or angry, your muscles tighten, that seemingly small contraction contributes to increased pain and then increased anxiety. And it can provoke other emotional pain like family and job-related issues that only compound the problem. You get the idea?

Long-term pain can actually affect your brain and your entire being. In its initial stages, an injury causes increased heart rate, prioritization of blood flow to the muscles, and other stress responses. Your body usually adapts to these changes and returns to normal fairly quickly. But chronic pain presents a different issue. Chronic, persistent pain leading to real psychological changes, pretty much like driving your car with the pedal to the metal for 1,000 miles. Over time, these stress responses impact your brain function, resulting in changes in behavior. Moreover, this chronic stress is not limited to psychological effects. Chronic pain and the resulting prolonged stress response can lead to heart issues, gastrointestinal changes, and more.

It probably goes without saying that the emotional toll of pain only increases with time. If your painful injury becomes chronic, those feelings of anger, anxiety and depression escalate. That is why it's so important to nip pain in the acute stage.

Quality of Life

The economic cost of chronic pain is important, but it pales in contrast to the uncountable losses to quality of life for those who cannot find a way around their pain. When someone becomes literally nonfunctional, not only can it mean job loss and economic insecurity, it can affect family relationships, friendships, and even the ability to perform the most basic tasks of daily life.

Not only are pain patients extremely susceptible to depression and anxiety, but their families are also at risk for the same mental health challenges. In one study, families of people with chronic pain said they felt "powerless, alienated, emotionally distressed, and isolated" in their efforts to nurture and sustain a family member with chronic pain.

One nationwide survey found that two-thirds of people with chronic pain expect to live with it for the rest of their lives. Wow! That sounds grim. As you may have already guessed, it does not have to be that way. Read on. You've no doubt already guessed some of the answers.

Other Costs of Pain

Beyond the emotional toll of something as simple as a broken leg, pain definitely extracts a financial toll on the individual and eventually on society.

Pain can be especially limiting for workers, no matter their job types. It's expensive in terms of the actual cost of treatment and the loss of productivity among those who suffer from long-term pain. Then there is the incalculable cost of loss of quality of life for those who suffer.

"If all chronic pain conditions were lumped together and considered to be a single disease, as many pain researchers view the problem, this aggregate would be the most common, disabling and expensive health problem in the world," says Daniel Clauw, M.D., director of the University of Michigan's Chronic Pain and Fatigue Research Center.

The Institute of Medicine (now known as the National Academy of Medicine) proclaimed chronic pain a public health problem more than five years ago, and the problem persists. These give us all the more reason to prevent acute pain from becoming chronic.

The Numbers

Here are some daunting U.S. numbers as reported by an American Health and Drug Benefits study:

- Approximately 100 million American adults have some type of pain condition. That is nearly half of the adult population of the country is in serious pain at any given moment.

Most of those people (89%) had reported pain for at least one year and 86% experienced pain two to three times a week or more.
- The estimated cost of chronic pain in medical expenses, lost wages and lost productivity is $635 billion annually.
- Chronic pain is on the rise. The 2008 Medical Expenditure Panel Survey (MEPS) found that the total number of adults with chronic back pain increased by an alarming 64% between 2000 and 2007. These increases have been linked to an aging population and the rising numbers of people with aggravating conditions such as obesity and diabetes.
- About 10% of American adults suffer from disabling chronic pain that prevents them from holding jobs.
- Those rising numbers were particularly noticeable in low-income individuals, certain ethnic groups, and women.
- Back pain is by far the most common source of chronic pain, but migraines and other headaches have a significant impact, as does knee pain.
- In the United States, an estimated 149 million work days are lost every year because of low back pain alone, with total costs estimated to be US $100 to 200 billion a year in lost wages and lower productivity.

The Pain of Poverty

The poorest members of our society are those most vulnerable to pain. Approximately 35% of people being treated for chronic back pain live at the poverty level ($12,670 for a single person). If we add those at the next rung on the poverty scale, those making under $25,000 a year, more than two-thirds of these sufferers are poor.

Poverty and Integrative Methods of Treatment for Pain

Recently I attended a seminar on the topic and was immediately struck by the lack of attention to the expense of the nonpharmacological treatments being advised to take the place of opioids. I watched the doctors on the panel enthusiastically promote acupuncture, yoga, chiropractic care, bio- feedback, massage, lidocaine patches, and TENS units. Yet, many of these treatments are not covered by most insurance plans and can be very expensive to pay for out of pocket. In the case of something like massage or acupuncture, it can cost well over $100 per visit. Since these therapies usually require multiple visits to achieve long-term outcomes, it can cost patients hundreds or thousands of dollars to cover the costs of such treatments. Considering that most people with disability live below the poverty level, many people with chronic pain may not be in a financial position to fund these alternative treatments—meaning they are basically unavailable to them.

Laura Kiesel, Harvard Health Letter 11-10-17

What You Need to Know:

- Pain takes an enormous financial and emotional toll on the lives of those in pain as well as their families, friends, and co-workers.
- About 100 million American adults suffer from pain. That's about half of the US adult population.
- Back pain is the most common type of long-term pain.
- Pain costs our economy about $635 billion a year in medical expenses and lost productivity and wages.
- The number of people with pain conditions have increased dramatically in the past few years. People of color, women, and low income are particularly vulnerable.
- Treatment of acute pain and prevention of digression to chronic pain are the clear ways to preventing these terrible losses.

CHAPTER 6
Conventional Medicine's Response to Pain

As you might imagine, conventional medicine does not offer many good answers to pain.

Some are moderately helpful, some worthless, some carry heavy side effects, and some are downright deadly.

Of course, it depends on where your pain is and how long you have had it. For example, surgery for back pain has been called sham surgery that rarely has benefits and may simply pave the way to additional surgeries and even eventual spinal fusion. However, surgery to replace a knee joint that is bone-on-bone can be a long-term solution for many people.

Aside from surgery and physical therapy, which is sometimes very effective for back pain and a few physical devices like TENS units, conventional medicine has little to offer chronic pain sufferers except pain-relieving drugs.

Tylenol

It seems so mild and innocuous. "My advice," your doctor says, "Take a couple of Tylenol and you'll be fine."

Chances are you won't be fine.

Acetaminophen, also known as paracetamol, is one of the generic names for Tylenol. It is the most widely used pain relief medication in the U.S. Nearly a quarter of us use it occasionally and some use it daily. It is also the leading cause of liver failure in the United States.

Even when taken according to doctor's orders, this over-the-counter NSAID (non-steroidal anti-inflammatory drug) can be deadly. It accounts for 100,000 calls to poison control centers annually and is responsible for about 60,000 emergency room visits and hundreds of deaths every year.

Even with its milder side effects, acetaminophen can cause gastric ulcers, heart attacks and strokes.

It's also added to more than 600 over-the-counter and prescription medications, so it's pretty much everywhere.

A 2015 British study warned that acetaminophen is more deadly than medical science once thought, even when taken at recommended dosages.

Other NSAIDS

I know, it is easy to think that over-the-counter pain relievers are safe, but that could not be farther from the truth.

Ibuprofen (most common brand name Motrin) and even aspirin seem mild and they work to relieve many minor aches and pains and reduce inflammation, whether they come from an acute injury or a long-standing problem. They work to bring down a fever. For decades, many of us have been told by our doctors to take a baby aspirin daily to prevent heart disease because it prevents blood clotting, a major factor in heart attacks and strokes.

Aspirin is a double-edged sword. Yes, there is strong evidence that supports the low-dose aspirin like those consumed by about one-third of Americans over 40 to reduce the risk of death from a heart attack or stroke.

But a recent pivotal study from George Washington Medical School concluded that the risk of serious gastrointestinal bleeding caused by aspirin was greater than its heart-protective benefits, calling into serious question the nearly universal aspirin recommendation.

In fact, those who took aspirin regularly had double the risk of major gastrointestinal bleeding than non-aspirin users, leading to more than 3,000 deaths a year. The risk increases as aspirin users age, rising to

5% of those over 85 experiencing major gastro-intestinal bleeds from aspirin usage with prescribed limits.

It is reasonable and prudent to conclude that long-term aspirin use for all purposes carries the same risk of gastrointestinal bleeding and potential death.

Beware if you take ibuprofen (Motrin or Advil) and naproxen (Aleve) for pain relief, you get the risk of acetaminophen and aspirin all rolled into one: increased risk of liver problems, heart attack and stroke, gastrointestinal bleeding, and kidney failure added in for good measure. WOW!

As far back as 2015, the U.S. Food and Drug Administration took the rare step of strengthening its warning of the increased risk of heart attack and stroke for long-term users of non-aspirin NSAIDS.

Of course, ibuprofen and naproxen are widely available over-the-counter. There are also prescription strength NSAIDS like celecoxib (Celebrex), diclofenac (Cataflam, Voltaren) and other NSAIDs that carry the same risks when used for extended periods of time.

Then There are Opioids...

You've heard about the opioid crisis. It is a national tragedy. It is a terrible downward spiral that often begins with a legal prescription for a chronic pain condition. These highly addictive drugs, even when taken at the proper dosages for legitimate pain, cause changes to the brain that spark a compulsive craving for more and more of the drug to experience the same relief (or high).

Even when used for legitimate reasons, such as short-term use for pain after surgery to address long-term intractable pain, opioids are so highly addictive that they can cause addiction even when used meticulously according to prescribed limits. Doctors are increasingly prescribing anti-inflammatories like NSAIDS right after surgery. While they are not without risk as you read in the paragraphs above, their risk is far less than with opioids.

An estimated 2 million Americans misuse opioids. In 2018, opioids were a factor in more than 46,000 deaths in the U.S. That includes more than 20,000 overdose deaths a year attributed to legally prescribed opioids and an additional 13,000 deaths are caused by illegal use, according to the Centers for Disease Control and Prevention. Drug overdoses are the #1 cause of accidental death in the U.S., according to the American Society of Addiction Medicine.

The most commonly prescribed opioids include oxycodone, fentanyl, buprenorphine, methadone, oxymorphone, hydrocodone, codeine, and morphine. Some other opioids, such as heroin, are illegal drugs to which many once-legal prescription opioid users turn when they can no longer obtain them legally.

Four companies that manufactured or distributed opioids and encouraged doctors to prescribe them were in the process of entering into a $26 billion settlement at this writing to protect them from further legal action from counties and cities ravaged by the opioid crisis. Another pharmaceutical company agreed to pay $8 billion in a similar settlement. Dozens of individual lawsuits and actions against pharmacies and other distributors are still active at this writing.

The *Washington Post* reported on Nov. 5, 2020:

> "In the opioid lawsuits, public officials have alleged that the opioid manufacturers, distributors and pharmacies knew, or should have known, that billions of the highly addictive pills they produce and sell for legitimate pain patients were siphoned off by fraudulent doctors, illegal pill mills and negligent pharmacies to people who abused the drugs."

> "More than 100 billion doses of two opioids—oxycodone and hydrocodone—flooded the country between 2006 and 2014, according to data obtained by the *Washington Post* in a lawsuit."

This may be more information than you need to know, but pay attention to the fact you should avoid opioids at all costs, no matter how severe your chronic pain might be.

Other Conventional Paths to Pain Relief

Cold or Heat Therapy: Simple application of an icepack or gel pack, or a heating pad can offer temporary relief.

Exercise: It might seem counterintuitive, but movement is often an effective pain management tool, especially for chronic pain that is caused by degenerative arthritis (osteoarthritis). It can help lubricate damaged joints and reduce inflammation if done gently. Swimming, walking, and bicycling can help.

Steroid Injections: Injecting steroids in hopes of dramatically reducing inflammation works well for some patients. In some people a single injection can erase the problem. Most people build up a tolerance for the steroids, requiring more frequent injections and dramatically raising the risk of heart disease.

Physical Therapy: We have mentioned physical therapy, which can be a blessing for many people with chronic pain, especially for people with back pain. Water therapy can be even more helpful. Many patients find relief from inversion chairs rather than inversion tables that potentially may put too much stress on ankle, knee, and hip joints.

TENS Unit: Transcutaneous electrical stimulation units are inexpensive and very effective for some people. The portable units have electrodes that deliver tiny electric shocks to painful areas and effectively block the pain signals to the brain. In serious cases, electrical stimulation units can be implanted surgically.

What You Need to Know:

- Conventional medicine has non-pharmaceutical ways of managing pain that range from the application of cold or heat to intensive physical therapy and electrical stimulation units. For some people, this may be all that is needed.
- Drug interventions are the most common way conventional medicine has to approach chronic pain ranging from over- the-counter medicines (NSAIDS non-steroidal anti-inflammatories) like aspirin, acetaminophen (Tylenol), ibuprofen (Motrin, Advil) and naproxen (Aleve) that can have deadly side effects to equally problematic prescription versions of these pain relievers.
- Prescriptions for opioids (oxycodone, fentanyl, buprenorphine, methadone, oxymorphone, hydrocodone, codeine, and morphine) are effective but inevitably lead to addiction with long-term use and require larger and larger doses to achieve the same level of pain relief.

CHAPTER 7
Natural Pain Relievers That Work

Pain does not have to become a way of life. Those of us who love natural living have no doubt discovered some natural pain relief and healing techniques for ourselves.

They range from chiropractic and osteopathy to massage, a broad variety of mind-body techniques to botanicals, essential oils, yoga, tai chi, meditation, and therapeutic modalities including music, dance, and pet therapy.

Most people who experience pain combine what works for them, sometimes drawing from conventional and unconventional methods.

Let us explore a few, again with an eye toward doing what it takes to keep acute pain from becoming chronic:

Body-Mind Therapies

A 2008 study from Northwestern University confirmed that people in chronic pain experience changes to the front region of the cortex which fail to deactivate from pain signals when it should. It is like the pain perception gets stuck pedal to the metal, stuck on full throttle, wearing out neurons and altering neural connections. Over time, this leads to measurable brain damage and cognitive and behavioral dysfunction.

What this means in simple terms is that the brain becomes incapable of turning off the pain signals. It almost inevitably leads to insomnia, anxiety, depression, and memory loss.

There are several techniques that help redirect and redefine pain signals to the brain. They won't cure the underlying cause of the pain, but they can help change the way your brain—and your mind and body respond to the pain stimulation. Among these techniques are:

- **Cognitive Behavioral Therapy** to help break the negative thought feedback loop that feeds the pain response.
- **Biofeedback** which uses sensors to help teach muscle relaxation and relieve pain. It is very effective for headaches.
- **Yogic Breathing Techniques** to promote relaxation, relieve muscle tension, and improve sleep.
- **Meditation**, especially mindfulness meditation, to retrain those potentially damaged neural pathways in the brain and even restructure the cortex to redirect pain sensations.

These modalities can all help you restore a sense of control over your body and turn down the "fight, flight or freeze" response, which can worsen chronic muscle tension and pain.

Chiropractic and Osteopathy

These are actually well validated and scientifically verified health care professions delivered by highly trained practitioners. Technically, they should not even be included in non-conventional modalities, but the truth is that many physicians mistrust and misunderstand them, so there are vast falsehoods surrounding both professions.

Chiropractors are trained to manipulate the musculoskeletal and nervous systems. Chiropractic adjustments can correct misalignments of the spine or other joints and have been proven to be very effective in relieving low back pain.

Osteopathic doctors, commonly called osteopaths, trigger the body's natural healing systems, often through manipulation of muscles and soft tissues.

While chiropractors are primarily focused on the joints and spine, osteopaths take on a more holistic approach targeting the entire body.

Acupuncture

Pain relief can be achieved by redirecting energy flows through meridians throughout the body with acupuncture. Famously, Chinese surgeons have used the ancient technique to perform surgery without anesthesia. An important 2017 review of studies published in the *Journal of Pain* concluded that acupuncture is effective in relieving chronic pain and the effects lasted at least a year.

Physical approaches

Having already mentioned professional manipulation like a chiropractor or an osteopath might offer, physical exercise can offer significant relief from chronic pain.

Yoga

Yoga, an ancient Indian tradition helps gently stretch and strengthen muscles and joints while providing overall relaxation. One study showed that a single 60-minute yoga class a week relieved pain and increased mobility better than standard pharmaceutical treatment. Another review of studies confirmed that yoga helps relieve low back pain in both the short-term and long-term. NOTE: The prolonged stretching involved in the practice of hatha yoga should always be slow, gentle and non-competitive. Some of today's more energetic forms of yoga can cause injury.

Walking

Many people with pain are reluctant to exercise and move for fear the pain will intensify. In fact, experts say movement actually helps relieve pain. Taking a brisk walk helps loosen and lubricate joints, especially for those with osteoarthritis and knee pain. It can also engage something called the exogenous opioid system. These are the good kind of feel-good brain chemicals—the natural pain relievers that the brain produces with exercise, sometimes known as the "runner's high."

Massage

Deep tissue massage may sometimes be painful because it helps release tight muscles, relieve impingement of joints and promote the release of pain-relieving brain chemicals, but the positive effects of deep tissue massage are well documented.

Botanicals and Supplements for Pain Relief

There are dozens of botanicals and supplements that can help with acute pain, although there are none that actually provide healing like the ones you'll read about in the next chapter. Most help relieve inflammation to one degree or another.

Here are a few:

- **Glucosamine and Chondroitin**: Can help relieve joint pain and improve movement. Research is mixed.
- **SAM-e (S-adenosyl-L-methionine)**: Works much like NSAIDS to relieve inflammation. Part of its effect on chronic pain may be that it helps relieve depression. Should not be taken with other antidepressants.
- **Willow Bark:** The source of salicins, the primary ingredient in aspirin. It works as a natural NSAID as well. Studies suggest it can be helpful in relieving headaches and back pain.
- **Capsaicin creams:** Works in an interesting way to interrupt pain signals to the neurons when applied to the skin. It is most effective when used for nerve pain, like diabetic peripheral neuropathy.
- **Ginger:** A powerful anti-inflammatory well researched for long-term pain relief. It has especially been used for rheumatoid arthritis
- **Devil's claw:** An African botanical used as an anti-inflammatory for knee and back pain.
- **Fish oil:** Two fatty acids, EPA and DHA, make up fish oil and both help reduce inflammation

although there is some evidence they may suppress immune function.
- **CBD Oil:** This hemp-derivative can be helpful for chronic pain and especially for cancer pain.
- **A variety of vitamins, including B6, B-complex, C, and D** may enhance the effects of other pain relievers. Research is mixed.

And there are many, many more, too many to detail in this space.

What You Need to Know:

A variety of integrative, complementary, and natural methods of pain relief are widely used and can be highly effective in providing short-term and long-term benefits without serious side effects.

The best-studied and effective therapies include:

- Acupuncture
- Exercise and especially gentle hatha yoga
- Cognitive Behavioral Therapy to reassign the brain's recognition of pain signals
- Chiropractic adjustment and/or osteopathy
- A broad variety of botanicals and other supplements that have varying degrees of success

CHAPTER 8
The Triple Superpower Botanical Combo for Natural Pain Relief

From Terry:

Injury is inevitable. It's all a part of life. With injury inevitably comes pain. Whether you've stubbed your toe, cut your finger in the kitchen, have a more serious and longer-term problem like arthritis due to aging, residual pain from an injury, or even cancer—you want relief and you want it fast.

Finding pain relief that is both fast-acting and safe has been nearly impossible until now.

A cutting-edge Indian study on a unique combination of curcumin, boswellia, and black sesame seed oil proves it, and opens up a whole new world for anyone who wants to relieve acute (sudden onset) pain.

Here's the superpower combo that can handle any kind of pain:

- Curcumin from turmeric (*curcuma longa*)
- Boswellia (*boswellia serrata*)
- Black sesame seed oil (*Sesamum indicum*)

Individually, each of these botanicals has a unique approach to pain. Combined, these three form a synergistic team that is unbeatable for its effectiveness and safety.

Let's take a look:

Curcumin is Gold

No doubt, you've heard of curcumin. If you love curry, you'll be familiar with turmeric, a vividly colored spice. Inside turmeric is a medicinal compound called curcumin, which is found in the rhizome (the stem of the plant found underground). Curcumin is responsible for the golden orange color of turmeric and is arguably the most powerful botanical medicine known today. However, there is very little curcumin in turmeric. I like to quote my friend, City of Hope Cancer Researcher Dr. Ajay Goel, who says, "Turmeric is the spice. Curcumin is the medicine."

Botanically known as *Curcuma longa*, curcumin is an antioxidant and anti-inflammatory from the ginger family with scientifically validated effectiveness against a broad range of chronic diseases, including heart disease, cancer, diabetes, Alzheimer's disease, and more. And, last but hardly least, it is a powerful ally against acute and chronic pain.

Curcumin is at least as effective as a broad variety of over-the-counter and prescription NSAIDS (remember those non-steroidal anti-inflammatory drugs like acetaminophen, ibuprofen, Celebrex, Bextra to relieve pain?) without the deadly side effects. In fact, it can be at least *eight* times more effective than Tylenol in reducing the emotional impacts of pain like we talked about in Chapter 5.

Inflammation causes pain, so if you relieve the inflammation, you relieve the pain. Like all NSAIDS, curcumin is a COX-2 inhibitor. In simple terms, this means it slows the inflammation-causing COX-2 enzyme. Unlike other NSAIDS, curcumin does NOT interrupt the COX-1 enzyme that protects the lining of the digestive tract and blood vessels. That means it doesn't cause the potentially deadly problems you'd find with acetaminophen, ibuprofen, Celebrex and other NSAIDS.

Not only does curcumin relieve inflammation, it can actually rebuild worn cartilage, restoring joints to their youthful flexibility. Add in the fact that curcumin is a potent antioxidant that can help repair oxidative damage caused by long-term inflammation and we've got a winner!

Sports medicine has been taking notice of curcumin for some time. In a Spanish double-blind, crossover trial, participants started taking curcumin two days before a physical workout and continued for three days after. Those taking curcumin noted moderate to large reductions in pain and slightly increased performance (due to the pain reduction). The exercises included gluteal stretches, squat jumps, and single-leg jumps, to get in a variety of controlled movements to replicate the wide range of motions that can cause pain during a workout.

Another study looked at the effects of curcumin and boswellia together for adult recreational cyclists. Those in the curcumin group reported feeling better than those in the placebo group and less stressed during training days that involved two hours of endurance cycling.

Researchers in this study noted that specific blood concentrations of curcumin were required to get consistent outcomes. I would say that the easiest way to guarantee results is to make sure you have a strong, clinically studied, enhanced absorption curcumin on board to begin with that has been tested for blood retention.

What Kind of Curcumin? Absorption is Key

If you've lived in India all of your life, you are probably consuming enough curcumin in your diet to get a medicinal result. Curcumin is only 2 to 5% of the total weight of turmeric. In a traditional Indian diet, fat helps with absorption. However, for the rest of us who haven't eaten turmeric daily for a lifetime, we need the medicinal component, curcumin.

Both turmeric and curcumin are difficult for the body to absorb. In fact, early research on curcumin necessitated that participants take 12 to 16 capsules a day to even reach measurable blood levels. This is impractical, which is why research now focuses on enhanced absorption curcumin. You need something that is scientifically proven, and both safe and effective to help curcumin absorb efficiently.

When you blend curcumin with the right ingredient, you don't need large doses to get results. The curcumin I prefer is blended with turmeric oils that offers a fuller spectrum of compounds from the turmeric plant and processed in a very specific way. In fact, this clinically studied curcumin known as BCM-95 is up to 700% better absorbed than plain curcumin and has much better blood retention time. Plus, the turmerones present in the oil provide their own anti-inflammatory and anticancer activity.

Boswellia serrata (Also Known as Frankincense)

Inflammation is not a singular activity in the body. In fact, there are a multitude of inflammatory pathways and one that is often overlooked and difficult to address is called the 5-lipoxygenase, or 5-LOX enzyme and pathway.

Boswellia is one of nature's most powerful anti-inflammatories. It is a specific inhibitor of 5-LOX, an enzyme that activates inflammation-inducing molecules called leukotrienes. Boswellia should be a favorite herb for anyone who experiences acute pain, which often has some level of 5-LOX activity.

Indian researchers made the impressive finding that people had a higher pain threshold and greater pain tolerance when taking boswellia. The reason the researchers wanted to explore this time-tested herbal medicine? Because we are still far from a breakthrough non-steroidal anti-inflammatory drug (NSAID) that doesn't adversely affect the gastrointestinal or cardiovascular systems. There is simply no risk-free pain reliever. For that matter, there are no other over-the-counter medicines that work on 5-LOX inflammation pathway. Even curcumin, one of my favorites, doesn't match boswellia on this specific pathway, which is why I recommend adding it to your triple superpower combo.

What Kind of Boswellia?

Commercially available boswellia varies greatly. The plant offers a number of compounds. Some, specifically acetyl-11-keto-boswellic acid (AKBA), are extremely beneficial, and most responsible for the extract's positive effects on reducing inflammation in the short-and long-term. However, another naturally occurring boswellia compound, beta-boswellic acid, is not beneficial. In fact, it actually promotes, rather than blocks, inflammation.

Researchers investigating the differences between boswellic acids have remarked that it could "activate the generation of (inflammation-promoting) arachidonic acid as well as activate 5-LOX and perpetuate the leukotrienes cascade of inflammation, rather than inhibit it, an effect opposite of what was intended." Of course, that's the last thing anyone wants when they're looking for pain relief.

That's why I prefer a specialized boswellia extract that reduces beta-boswellic acids to less than 5%. Think of the process as being similar to decaffeinating coffee—there's still a very small percentage of caffeine left, but not enough to cause jitteriness for most people. Plus, at the end of the process, you still have real coffee, not something artificial or cooked up in a lab. The same is true with boswellia—you can filter out the "bad" and keep the good. Ultimately, this maximizes the extract's potency, because it does not have to fight against itself to reduce pain and muscle damage caused by inflammation. But just as importantly, you still have natural boswellia. The extract I recommend is also standardized for a minimum of 70 percent boswellic acids, emphasizing only those that increase its effectiveness, including at least 10 percent AKBA. Unstandardized extracts can provide as little as one percent AKBA and they don't filter out beta-boswellic acid.

Black Sesame (*Sesamum indicum*) Seed Oil

Sesame seed oil is something we may not normally think of as an herbal medicine, but there are reasons why we should.

Sesame seed oil contains compounds that have been shown to have anti-inflammatory effects for synovial (joint) tissue in cases of rheumatoid arthritis

(RA). Scientific research shows that it reduces the activity of TNF-a, inflammatory proteins called cytokines that are responsible for much of the damage caused by RA.

In scientific studies of osteoarthritis, too, sesame seed compounds have shown joint protecting actions. Even just one of the compounds in sesame seed, sesamin, can help increase type II collagen and prostaglandins and prevent the breakdown of beneficial fatty acids that keep joints healthy and stop painful damage.

Other work with sesame seed components, especially sesamin, has found the same results; this botanical preserves the cushioning elements of joints because of its specific anti-inflammatory strengths.

In clinical research, supplementation with sesame seed has been shown to reduce inflammatory markers, pain scores, and symptoms in patients with knee osteoarthritis.

Additionally, sesame seed appears to help other nutrients absorb more effectively, having a synergistic effect on, and helping concentrate levels of vitamin E tocopherols, vitamin C, and vitamin K.

Other general research with sesame seed has found that it helps control the ratio of omega-3 and omega-6 fatty acids, helps balance cholesterol levels, and has overall immune, cardiovascular, and DNA-protective actions.

Triple Superpower

The combination of absorption enhancement and anti-inflammatory power is something that attracted Indian researchers to sesame seed oil in their efforts to find an effective and fast pain-relieving combination that included curcumin and boswellia.

They chose to use black sesame seed as a source of the oil, because black sesame seeds are higher in beneficial lignans like sesamin and valuable phenolic compounds than white sesame seeds.

With that in mind, the curcumin and boswellia combination in this study was specially emulsified in black sesame seed oil, which helps disperse these fat-soluble herbs in the intestines, where they can be absorbed into the bloodstream for optimal pain fighting ability. Additionally, black sesame seed oil also has a long history of use in Ayurvedic practice as an anti-inflammatory and may actually help raise levels of glutathione—the body's own master antioxidant, disease fighter, and detoxifier.

Beginning on day one of the study, the synergistic herbal combo matched acetaminophen in reducing pain intensity and pain magnitude, holding steady all the way through day seven, the conclusion of the trial. Additionally, the botanical combination was 8.5 times better than acetaminophen at reducing the emotional distress and unpleasantness associated with pain that *increases* the perceptions of pain.

The fact that these herbal ingredients had this effect is not surprising. Curcumin alone has been shown to be equal to prescription medication in alleviating symptoms of depression. These symptoms have an inflammatory component, just as much as they have a biochemical one; with three powerful anti-inflammatories working through a multitude of pathways, they are more active in addressing that aspect of pain better.

In fact, there is a growing body of research that shows that because of the way acetaminophen works in the brain, it actually reduces a person's capacity to feel empathy for another's pain or joy. In fact, some researchers have called acetaminophen a "social analgesic" because of the way it cuts off the ability to socially connect at a basic, human level with other people. When you consider that over 600 medicines include acetaminophen, it creates a frightening picture of the way this drug can emotionally separate us from one another.

Admittedly, the emotional distress of pain is a broad category. It's tough to put a box around how we perceive pain. In some cases, having a sense of 'control' over how you feel can lessen its overall impact, if not its intensity.

For example, research shows that even though the level of pain may be the same, when people felt like they had some control over pain, if they felt less helpless, there was less emotional suffering. It seems that this herbal combination allowed people to feel they were still making some choice over how they felt, while not shutting down healthy connections in the mind that relate to empathy and goodwill.

Curcumin, Boswellia, and Black Sesame Oil

THE BEST CHOICE FOR FIGHTING ACUTE PAIN

- Modulates multiple inflammatory pathways in the body, including COX-2 and 5-LOX
- Does NOT cause liver damage, stomach upset, gastric ulcers, high blood pressure, kidney damage, or risk of heart attack
- Works as fast as acetaminophen for acute pain when emulsified in black sesame oil, a traditional Ayurvedic botanical recommended by practitioners for centuries

THE FORMULA I SUGGEST IS A 500 MG PROPRIETARY COMPLEX CONTAINING:

- Black Sesame (*Sesamum indicum*) Seed Oil
- Curcumin (*Curcuma longa*) Rhizome Extract (BCM-95®/ Curcugreen®) enhanced with turmeric essential oil and standardized for curcuminoid complex (curcumin, demethoxycurcumin and bisdemethoxycurcumin)

- Boswellia (*Boswellia serrata*) Gum Resin Extract (BOS-10™) standardized to contain 70% Total Organic and Boswellic Acids with AKBA 10%, with 5% beta-boswellic acids

CHAPTER 9
Doc to Doc

Dear Doctor,

Like most books, this book is copyrighted. However, the information presented here is so important to your patients' health and to your scientific knowledge that we have urged our readers to copy this chapter and give it to you in hopes that this brief summary of a combination of three botanicals will help you recognize its effectiveness in safely and effectively treating acute and chronic pain.

In the interest of respecting your time, I ask you to read these few brief pages.

First, let me briefly introduce myself:

I am Jan McBarron, M.D., N.D. With over thirty years in private medical practice. My clinical approach remains to offer patients the best in complimentary medicine. A combination of traditional and natural medicine often provides the most benefit and best outcome for the patient. Too often physicians as well as patients feel these two modalities are mutually exclusive, its either "real" medicine or "alternative". Drugs are readily accepted while herbs are often dismissed, and their science ignored.

I first wrote about curcumin (*Curcuma longa*) in 2012 in my book, *Curcumin: The 21st Century Cure*. As I researched the botanical and prescribed it in my practice, I was deeply impressed with its effectiveness in treating a broad spectrum of conditions, including acute and chronic pain.

In the eight years since *The 21st Century Cure* was published, there has been a greater body of research into curcumin's effectiveness and exciting new research that confirms the synergistic pain-relieving properties of curcumin when combined with boswellia (*Boswellia serrata*) and black sesame seed oil (*Sesamum indicum*).

While my current book, *Relieve Pain Without Side Effects*, addresses this combination for acute pain relief, in my experience, it is just as effective in addressing chronic pain.

The following is a brief overview of the mechanism of action for each of the three botanicals:

Curcumin

Curcumin, the rhizome of the turmeric plant, is a potent antioxidant and anti-inflammatory from the ginger family with scientifically validated effectiveness against a broad range of chronic diseases, including heart disease, cancer, diabetes, Alzheimer's disease, and more. In addition, it is a powerful ally against acute and chronic pain.

Curcumin is at least as effective as a broad variety of over-the-counter and prescription NSAIDS without the deadly side effects. In fact, it can be at least eight times more effective than Tylenol in reducing the emotional impact of pain, including anxiety and depression.

Like all NSAIDS, curcumin is a COX-2 inhibitor. Unlike other NSAIDS, curcumin does NOT interrupt the COX-1 enzyme that protects the lining of the digestive tract and blood vessels. That means it does not cause the potentially fatal gastrointestinal side effects found with usage of acetaminophen, ibuprofen, Celebrex, and other NSAIDS.

Not only does curcumin relieve inflammation and acute pain as well as osteoarthritis and rheumatoid arthritis pain, several studies, including a highly credible German one, show curcumin helps rebuild worn cartilage.

Curcumin is also a potent antioxidant that helps repair oxidative damage caused by long-term inflammation. Sports medicine has been taking notice of curcumin for some time. In a Spanish double-blind, crossover trial, participants started taking curcumin two days before a physical workout and continued for three days after. Those taking curcumin noted moderate to large reductions in pain and slightly increased performance (due to the pain reduction). The exercises included gluteal stretches, squat jumps, and single-leg jumps, to get in a variety of controlled movements to replicate the wide range of motions that can cause pain during a workout.

What kind of curcumin? Curcumin is not easily bioabsorbable. The curcumin I prefer is blended with turmeric oil that offers a fuller spectrum of compounds from the turmeric plant and processed in an extremely specific way. In fact, this clinically studied curcumin formulation known as BCM-95, is up to 700% better absorbed than ordinary curcumin and has much better blood retention time. Plus, the turmerones present in the oil provide their own anti-inflammatory and anticancer activity.

Boswellia serrata (commonly known as frankincense)

Inflammation is not a singular activity in the body. In fact, there are a multitude of inflammatory pathways and one often over-looked and difficult to address is the 5-lipoxygenase, or 5-LOX enzyme pathway.

Boswellia is one of nature's most powerful anti-inflammatories.

It is a specific inhibitor of 5-LOX, an enzyme that activates inflammation-inducing molecules called leukotrienes. Boswellia should be seriously considered for anyone who experiences acute pain, which often has some level of 5-LOX activity.

Indian research yielded the impressive finding that people had a higher pain threshold and greater pain tolerance when taking boswellia. What was the impetus for researchers to explore this time-tested herbal medicine?

Because as health care providers, we remain far from a breakthrough non-steroidal anti-inflammatory drug (NSAID) that does not adversely affect the gastrointestinal or cardiovascular systems. There is simply no risk-free pain reliever. For that matter, there are no other over-the-counter medicines that work on 5-LOX inflammation pathway. Even curcumin, one of my favorites, does not match boswellia on this specific pathway, which is why I recommend including it in a triple superpower formulation.

Another study looked at the effects of curcumin and boswellia together for adult recreational cyclists. Those in the curcumin group reported feeling better than those in the placebo group and less stressed during training days that involved two hours of endurance cycling.

Researchers in this study noted that specific blood concentrations of curcumin were required to get consistent outcomes. The easiest way to guarantee results is to start with a strong, clinically studied, enhanced absorption curcumin that has been tested for blood retention.

What kind of boswellia? Commercially available boswellia varies greatly. The plant offers several compounds. Some, specifically acetyl-11-keto-boswellic acid (AKBA), are *extremely* beneficial, and largely responsible for the extract's positive effects on reducing inflammation in the short and long term. However, another naturally occurring boswellia compound, beta-boswellic acid, is not beneficial. In fact, it actually *promotes*, rather than blocks, inflammation.

Researchers investigating the differences between boswellic acids have remarked that it could "activate the generation of (inflammation-promoting) arachidonic acid as well as activate 5-LOX and perpetuate the leukotrienes cascade of inflammation, rather than inhibit it, an effect opposite of what was intended." Of course, that's the last thing we want for pain relief. For that reason, I recommend a specialized boswellia extract that reduces beta-boswellic acids to less than 5%. The extract should also be standardized for a minimum of 70 percent boswellic acids, emphasizing only those that increase its effectiveness, including at least 10 percent AKBA. Unstandardized extracts can provide as little as one percent AKBA and they do not filter out beta-boswellic acid.

Black sesame seed oil (sesamum indicum)

The final natural ingredient of this synergistic triad is black sesame seed oil.

Sesame seed oil contains anti-inflammatory compounds that promote synovial tissue health in cases of rheumatoid arthritis (RA). Research shows that it reduces the activity of TNF-a, inhibiting cytokines that are responsible for much of the damage caused by RA.

In scientific studies of osteoarthritis also, sesame seed compounds have shown joint protecting actions. Even just one of the compounds in sesame seed, sesamin, can help increase type II collagen and prostaglandins and prevent the breakdown of beneficial fatty acids that keep joints healthy and stop painful damage.

In clinical research, supplementation with sesame seed has been shown to reduce inflammatory markers, pain scores and symptoms in patients with osteoarthritis of the knee.

Additionally, sesame seed appears to help other nutrients absorb more effectively, having a synergistic effect on, and helping concentrate levels of vitamin E tocopherols, vitamin C, and vitamin K.

Triple Superpower

The combination of absorption enhancement and anti-inflammatory power is something that attracted Indian researchers to sesame seed oil in their work on a pain-relieving combination that included curcumin and boswellia.

They chose to use black sesame seed as a source of the oil, because black sesame seeds are higher in beneficial lignans like sesamin and valuable phenolic compounds than white sesame seeds.

With that in mind, the curcumin and boswellia combination in this study was specially emulsified in black sesame seed oil, which helps disperse these fat-soluble herbs in the intestines, where they can be absorbed into the bloodstream for optimal pain fighting ability. Additionally, black sesame seed oil also has a long history of use in Ayurvedic practice as an anti-inflammatory and is thought to help increase levels of glutathione—the body's own master antioxidant, disease fighter, and detoxifier.

Beginning on day one of the study, the synergistic herbal combo matched acetaminophen in reducing pain intensity and pain magnitude, holding steady all the way through day seven, the conclusion of the trial. Additionally, the botanical combination was 8.5 times better than acetaminophen at reducing the emotional distress and unpleasantness associated with pain that *increases* the perceptions of pain.

Curcumin, Boswellia, And Black Sesame Oil

The Best Choice for Fighting Acute Pain:

- Modulates multiple inflammatory pathways in the body, including COX-2 and 5-LOX
- Does NOT cause liver damage, nausea, gastritis, gastric ulcers, high blood pressure, kidney damage, or risk of heart attack
- Works as fast as acetaminophen for acute pain when emulsified in black sesame oil, a traditional Ayurvedic botanical recommended by practitioners for centuries

In conclusion...

Having extensively reviewed the literature, the formula I recommend is a 500 mg proprietary complex containing:

- Black Sesame (*Sesamum indicum*) Seed Oil
- Curcumin (*Curcuma longa*) Rhizome Extract (BCM- 95®/Curcugreen®) enhanced with turmeric essential oil and standardized for curcuminoid complex (curcumin, demethoxycurcumin and bisdemethoxycurcumin)
- Boswellia (*Boswellia serrata*) Gum Resin Extract (BOS- 10™) standardized to contain 70% Total Organic and Boswellic Acids with AKBA 10%, with 5% beta-boswellic acids

While this botanical combination is safe and effective against acute pain, I am medically confident it will be just as effective for my patients with chronic pain.

—Jan McBarron M.D., N.D.

Key References

Buhrmann C, Honarvar A et al. Herbal Remedies as Potential in Cartilage Tissue Engineering: An Overview of New Therapeutic Approaches and Strategies. Molecules. 2020 Jul 6;25(13):3075.

Fernandez-Lazaro D, Mielgo-Ayuso J et al. Modulation of Exercise-Induced Muscle Damage, Inflammation, and Oxidative Markers by Curcumin Supplementation in a Physically Active Population: A Systematic Review. Nutrients. 2020 Feb; 12(2): 501.

Shaheen H and Alsenosy AA, Nuclear Factor Kappa B Inhibition as a Therapeutic Target of Nutraceuticals in Arthritis, Osteoarthritis, and Related Inflammation. Bioactive Food as Dietary Interventions for Arthritis and Related Inflammatory Diseases (Second Edition), Academic Press, 2019.

Hsu DZ, Chu, PY. Daily sesame oil supplement attenuates joint pain by inhibiting muscular oxidative stress in osteoarthritis rat model, The Journal of Nutritional Biochemistry 29, October 2015.

Rudrappa GH, Chakravarthi PT et al. Efficacy of high-dissolution turmeric- sesame formulation for pain relief in adult subjects with acute musculoskeletal pain compared to acetaminophen. Medicine (Baltimore). 2020 Jul 10; 99(28).

References

Chapter 1

Book reference:

Ingraham PS. Sensitization in Chronic Pain: Pain itself can change how pain works, resulting in more pain with less provocation. PainScience.com. painscience.com/articles/sensitization.php

Publications:

Zhu X, Li Q. Curcumin Alleviates Neuropathic Pain by Inhibiting p300/ CBP Histone Acetyltransferase Activity-Regulated Expression of BDNF and Cox-2 in a Rat Model. PLoS One. 2014; 9(3): e91303.

Babu A, Prasanth KG et al. Effect of curcumin in mice model of vincristine-induced neuropathy. Pharmaceutical Biology. Volume 53, 201, Issue 6.

Sun J , Chen F. Role of curcumin in the management of pathological pain. Phytomedicine. 2018 Sep 15;48:129–40.

Chapter 2

Zhang Z, Leong D. Curcumin slows osteoarthritis progression and relieves osteoarthritis-associated pain symptoms in a post-traumatic osteoarthritis mouse model. Arthritis Res Ther. 2016 Jun 3;18(1):128.

Zhang X, Guan Z. Curcumin Alleviates Oxaliplatin-Induced Peripheral Neuropathic Pain through Inhibiting Oxidative Stress-Mediated Activation of NF-kB and Mitigating Inflammation. Biol Pharm Bull. 2020 Feb 1;43(2):348–55.

Majeed M, Mjeed S et al. A pilot, randomized, double-blind, placebo- controlled trial to assess the safety and efficacy of a novel Boswellia serrata extract in the management of osteoarthritis of the knee. Phytother Res. 2019 May;33(5):1457–68.

Kimatkar N, Thawani V et al. Efficacy and tolerability of Boswellia serrata extract in treatment of osteoarthritis of knee—a randomized double blind placebo controlled trial. Phytomed. 2003 Jan; 10(1):3–7

REFERENCES

Gupta Pk, Samarakoon SMS et al. Clinical evaluation of Boswellia serrata (Shallaki) resin in the management of Sandhivata (osteoarthritis). Ayu. 2011 Oct–Dec; 32(4): 478–82.

Sumantran VN, Joshi AK et al. Antiarthritic activity of a standardized, multiherbal, Ayurvedic formulation containing Boswellia serrata: in vitro studies on knee cartilage from osteoarthritis patients. Phytother. Res. 2011 Sep;25(9):1375–80.

Rudrappa GH, Chakravarthi PT. Efficacy of high-dissolution turmeric-sesame formulation for pain relief in adult subjects with acute musculoskeletal pain compared to acetaminophen: A randomized controlled study. Medicine (Baltimore). 2020 Jul 10;99(28):e20373.

Haroyan A, Mukichyan V et al. Efficacy and safety of curcumin and its combination with boswellic acid in osteoarthritis: a comparative, randomized, double-blind, placebo-controlled study. BMC Complement Altern Med. 2018; 18: 7.

Chapter 3

Xiao L, Ding M. et al. Curcumin alleviates lumbar radiculopathy by reducing neuroinflammation, oxidative stress and nocioceptive factors. Eur Cell Mater. 2017 May 9;33:279–93.

Sun J. Chen F. Role of curcumin in the management of pathological pain. Phytomedicine. 2018 Sept 15;48:129–40.

Zhao X, Xu Y et al. Curcumin exerts antinociceptive effects in a mouse model of neuropathic pain: descending monoamine system and opioid receptors are differentially involved. Neuropharmacology. 2012 Feb;62(2):843–54.

Hsu CC, Huang HC et al. Sesame oil improves functional recovery by attenuating nerve oxidative stress in a mouse model of acute peripheral nerve injury: role of Nrf-2. J Nutr Biochem. 2016 Dec;38:102–106.

Chapter 4

Prabhavathi K, Chandra USJ et al. A randomized, double blind, placebo controlled, cross over study to evaluate the analgesic activity of Boswellia serrata in healthy volunteers using mechanical pain model. Indian J Pharam- col. 2014 Sep–Oct; 46(5): 475–79.

Edwards RR, Doleys DM, Fillingim RB, Lowery D. Ethnic differences in pain tolerance: clinical implications in a chronic pain population. Psychosom Med. 2001;63:316–23.

Chapter 5

Scientific papers:

Pasquale M. The Emotional Impact of the Pain Experience: Adapted from a presentation at the SLE Workshop at Hospital for Special Surgery on December 18, 2008. hss.edu/conditions_emotional-impact-pain-experience.asp

Institute of Medicine. Relieving Pain in America: A Blueprint for Transforming Prevention, Care, Education, and Research. Washington, DC: The National Academies Press; 2011. books.nap.edu/openbook.php?record_id=13172&page=17. Accessed November 10, 2014.

American Health and Drug Benefits onlineahdbonline.com/articles/2003-socioeconomic-burden-of-chronic-pain

Studies:

Baliki MN, Geha PY et al. Beyond Feeling: Chronic Pain Hurts the Brain, Disrupting the Default-Mode Network Dynamics. J Neurosci. 2008 Feb 6; 28(6): 1398–1403.

Johannes CB, Le TK, Zhou X, et al. The prevalence of chronic pain in United States adults: results of an Internet-based survey. J Pain. 2010;11:1230–39.

Smith M, Davis MA, Stano M, Whedon JM. Aging baby boomers and the rising cost of chronic back pain: secular trend analysis of longitudinal Medical Expenditures Panel Survey data for years 2000 to 2007. J Manipulative Physiol Ther. 2013;36:2–11.

Chapter 6

Roberts E, Nunes VD et al. Paracetamol: not as safe as we thought? A systematic literature review of observational studies. Ann Rheum Dis. 2016 Mar;75(3): 552–59.

Fernandez-Jimenez R, Wang TJ et al. Low-Dose Aspirin for Primary Prevention of Cardiovascular Disease: Use Patterns and Impact Across Race and Ethnicity in the Southern Community Cohort Study. Journal of the Ameri- can Heart Association. 2019;8:24.

Chapter 7

Vickers AJ, Vertosick EA et al. Acupuncture for Chronic Pain: Update of an Individual Patient Data Meta-Analysis. Critical Reviews. 2018; 9:5.

Cramer H, Lauche R et al. A systematic review and meta-analysis of yoga for low back pain. Clin J Pain. 2013 May;29(5):450–60.

REFERENCES

Zeidan F, Martucci KT et al. Brain Mechanisms Supporting the Modulation of Pain by Mindfulness Meditation. J Neurosci. 2011 Apr 6; 31(14): 5540–48.

Chapter 9

Buhrmann C, Honarvar A et al. Herbal Remedies as Potential in Cartilage Tissue Engineering: An Overview of New Therapeutic Approaches and Strategies. Molecules. 2020 Jul 6;25(13):3075.

Fernandez-Lazaro D, Mielgo-Ayuso J et al. Modulation of Exercise-Induced Muscle Damage, Inflammation, and Oxidative Markers by Curcumin Supplementation in a Physically Active Population: A Systematic Review. Nutrients. 2020 Feb; 12(2): 501.

Shaheen H and Alsenosy AA, Nuclear Factor Kappa B Inhibition as a Therapeutic Target of Nutraceuticals in Arthritis, Osteoarthritis, and Related Inflammation. Bioactive Food as Dietary Interventions for Arthritis and Related Inflammatory Diseases (Second Edition), Academic Press, 2019.

Hsu DZ, Chu, PY. Daily sesame oil supplement attenuates joint pain by inhibiting muscular oxidative stress in osteoarthritis rat model, The Journal of Nutritional Biochemistry 29, October 2015.

Rudrappa GH, Chakravarthi PT et al. Efficacy of high-dissolution turmeric-sesame formulation for pain relief in adult subjects with acute musculoskeletal pain compared to acetaminophen. Medicine (Baltimore). 2020 Jul 10; 99(28).

About the Authors

Terry Lemerond

Terry Lemerond is a natural health expert with over 50 years of experience helping people live healthier, vibrant lives. A much sought-after speaker and accomplished author, Terry shares his wealth of experience and knowledge in health and nutrition through his educational programs. They include the *Terry Talks Nutrition* website—TerryTalksNutrition.com— newsletters, podcasts, webinars, personal speaking engagements, and his popular, weekly radio show. His books include *Seven Keys to Vibrant Health*, *Seven Keys to Unlimited Personal Achievement,* and *50+ Natural Health Secrets Proven to Change Your Life*. Terry continues to author and co-author books with dedication, energy, and zeal around his ongoing mission — to help everyone improve their health.

Jan McBarron

Jan McBarron M.D., N.D., has been called "Doc" for more than thirty years. Initially she earned a BS in Nursing. Subsequently while working night shift as a nurse, she attended Drexel University School of Medicine in Philadelphia and earned her M.D/, Medical Doctorate.

In 1987, she opened her private medical practice, specializing in Medical Bariatrics in Georgia. While working full time, she studied natural medicine and earned her ND, Naturopathic Doctorate.

She maintains that most physicians and patients believe in either standard allopathic (MD), or alternative wellness medicine (ND). Having dual degrees allows her to practice from the best of both worlds, it is what "Doc" calls true complementary medicine. Her husband, Duke Liberatore, founded and grew a highly successful chain of health food stores. In 1993, they started Duke & The Doctor health talk radio. The broadcast aired every weekday for two hours, was nationally syndicated. and heard by millions in over 150 cities. The show garnered numerous awards including "Best Health Talk Show in the Nation," and the "Top 100 Best Talk Shows" by the prestigious Talkers Magazine based in New York. The show holds the distinct honor of being the first talk radio ever to broadcast from the Rock 'n Roll Hall of Fame. The couple discontinued their show upon the sale of Duke's stores in 2014. In addition, Doc has received many accolades over her career.

They have all been special to her but the ones she holds dear include Girl Scout Women of Achievement, Top Doctors in Atlanta, Top Doctor in Columbus, Readers' Choice Best in Weight Loss (every year for 30 years), Distinguished Alumni for Entrepreneurship from Drexel University, and 2010 Clinician of The Year.

In 2018, Duke and Doc moved closer to friends and family in Nevada. Doc gave up seeing patients one on one but believes she can reach many more people thru the Internet, writing, and public speaking. She continues to educate people thru her blogs and website Dr.JanMcBarron.com, as well as social media. In addition, she serves on the Scientific Board of Advisors to supplement companies and writes for many publications including Good Health Magazine.

She has written many books on health, nutrition and weight loss and is a recognized author on Amazon.

More about TTN Publishing, LLC
Everyone has the same desire:
a vibrant, healthy life!

TTN Publishing exists to provide educational information anyone can use to understand how herbs and botanical medicines play a vital role in optimal health. From a stomach ache to a life-threatening disease, even cancer, the plant kingdom has safe, effective phytonutrients and answers for healthy living.

Author and health pioneerTerry Lemerond brings his vast knowledge of plant medicines combined with cutting edge research from today's top scientists and doctors directly to consumers.

Each TTN Publishing, LLC book is crafted to provide the necessary basic information and recommendations for how botanicals can be used in practical ways to fight disease and improve the path to healthy living.

Education, information, scientific validation, and common sense are a part of every TTN Publishing endeavor. There are many books to come, so stay connected! With 80 percent of the world's population depending on plant medicines, you can join in the knowledge and wisdom available to meet your health goals.

Welcome to TTN Publishing!

We'd love to hear from you!
info@ttnpublishing.com
TTNPublishing.com
Would you like to be one of the first to know the latest updates on Terry's books?

- Learn more about his background and new books
- See photos, videos, and the latest news
- Listen to Terry's radio show, including archived programs on a multitude of subjects
- Sign up for a free weekly email newsletter and educational webinar notices

It's all available at TerryTalksNutrition.com

Don't forget to connect at:
facebook.com/TerryTalksNutrition

- Visit and follow Terry's author page on Amazon -amazon.com/author/terrylemerond

Share your good thoughts with other health seekers and leave a book review!

Share this exciting news!

If you appreciated this book, please let others know.

- Pick up another copy and share with a friend
- Talk about it on social media
- Write a review on your blog or website
- Recommend this book to friends and family

Thank you for being a true health seeker!
TTN Publishing, LLC

Made in the USA
Columbia, SC
25 August 2022